How to Improve Your Memory Fast

324 Effective Tips To Sharpen Your Memory And Boost Brainpower

ADAM COLTON

Published by BizMove
www.bizmove.com

ISBN: 1979466467
ISBN- 978-1979466462

Table of Contents

1. Memory Loss Fact Sheet

Many people worry about becoming forgetful. They think forgetfulness is the first sign of Alzheimer's disease. But not all people with memory problems have Alzheimer's.

Other causes for memory problems can include aging, medical conditions, emotional problems, mild cognitive impairment, or another type of dementia.

Age-Related Changes in Memory

Forgetfulness can be a normal part of aging. As people get older, changes occur in all parts of the body, including the brain. As a result, some people may notice that it takes longer to learn new things, they don't remember information as well as they did, or they lose things like their glasses. These usually are signs of mild forgetfulness, not serious memory problems, like Alzheimer's disease.

Mary's Story

Mary couldn't find her car keys. She looked on the hook just inside the front door. They weren't there. She searched in her purse. No luck. Finally, she found them on her desk. Yesterday, she forgot her neighbor's name. Her memory was playing tricks on her. She was starting to worry about it.

She decided to see her doctor. After a complete check-up, her doctor said that Mary was fine. Her forgetfulness was just a normal part of getting older. The doctor suggested that Mary take a class, play cards with friends, or help out at the local school to sharpen her memory.

Memory Loss Related to Medical Conditions

Certain medical conditions can cause serious memory problems. These problems should go away once a person gets treatment. Medical conditions that may cause memory problems include:

- Tumors, blood clots, or infections in the brain
- Some thyroid, kidney, or liver disorders
- Chronic alcoholism
- Head injury, such as a concussion from a fall or accident
- Medication side effects
- Not eating enough healthy foods, or too few vitamins and minerals in a person's body (like vitamin B12)

A doctor should treat serious medical conditions like these as soon as possible.

Al's Story

Al didn't know what was happening. He was having a hard time remembering things. He wasn't eating or sleeping well and didn't want to see friends. He was confused and irritable.

His wife was worried. She took him to the doctor. It turned out that Al was having a bad reaction to one of his medicines. Once his doctor changed his medicine, Al felt more like himself.

Memory Loss Related to Emotional Problems

Emotional problems, such as stress, anxiety, or depression, can make a person more forgetful and can be mistaken for dementia. For instance, someone who has recently retired or who is coping with the death of a spouse, relative, or friend may feel sad, lonely, worried, or bored. Trying to deal with these life changes leaves some people feeling confused or forgetful.

The confusion and forgetfulness caused by emotions usually are temporary and go away when the feelings fade. Emotional problems can be eased by supportive friends and family, but if these feelings last for a long time, it is important to get help from a doctor or counselor. Treatment may include counseling, medication, or both. Being active and learning new skills can also help a person feel better and improve his or her memory.

Gloria's Story

Gloria was feeling sad all the time. She just wanted to sleep all day and night. She was becoming really forgetful, too. Gloria's nephew Bob was afraid something was very wrong. He took her to see a doctor. The doctor said she had depression and needed to take medicine and see a counselor.

After 3 months, Bob could see the change in his aunt. She was eating and sleeping better. Gloria was spending more time with friends and doing volunteer work.

2. 324 Effective Tips To Sharpen Your Memory And Boost Brainpower

Memory can be defined as simply a person's ability to store, retain and recall information such as personal experiences. Of course, memory may be easy to understand but it's not exactly easy to remember everything. Some people have trouble with memory, and the tips in this article below can help you remember.

1. One of the best ways to store new information in memory is to relate it to something else that you are already familiar with. Creating a logical link between the new information and something else that you already know will increase your chances of being able to successfully recall that information later. The link you create functions as a trigger to recall the new information.

2. If you find yourself having difficulty remembering some things, try to use acronyms or tricks called mnemonics to help you remember. An example of this is to use Roy G. Biv to remember the colors of the rainbow as red, orange, yellow, green, blue,

indigo and violet. These types of tricks can really improve your memory.

3. Memory is just like the muscles in your body, if you don't use it, you'll lose it. A way to keep your memory active is to change up your brain's routine every so often. By doing the same activities over and over, you don't give your memory a chance to learn something new. By doing this, you will eventually start to lose your memory. Work your memory out by doing different activities including brain-stimulating activities in order to get the most out of your memory.

4. One of the most popular ways to commit information to your long-term memory is to utilize one of many different mnemonic devices. Mnemonic devices are similar to how writers use shorthand when writing. If you can associate a common item or word with something you want to remember, you create a roadmap in your brain to retrieve the information.

5. Visualizing yourself recalling information is actually a great way in which you can work to recall information. You are basically training your brain to be able to memorize items when you foresee yourself dipping into that memory bank to pull them out at a later date. Think of it like visualizing

your hand turning a doorknob before you actually turn it.

6. Eat more onions to improve your memory. A few studies have isolated fisetin to be of great benefit in improving the long term memory. You can find beneficial levels of fisetin in onions, strawberries, mangos and other plants. It also is a strong antioxidant so it will deliver other benefits to your body as well.

7. If you find that your memory has deteriorated drastically in a short period of time, it is important that you see your doctor right away. Sudden memory loss could be a sign of a more serious medical condition, such as Dementia or Alzheimer's Disease, which can effect people of all ages.

8. To better commit names to memory, repeat a person's name after an introduction, and try to come up with something about the person that might help you remember his or her name. If you meet a Bob who mentions that he enjoys fishing, you might associate his name with a bobber like those used on a fishing line, for instance.

9. If you have a hard time memorizing things, it is wise to try not to learn too many new things at the same time. Wait until you have fully memorized a

piece of information before moving on to the other. Learning many things at the same time will just make everything scramble in your brain.

10.   Try visual association to help with memory issues. The technique basically entails putting a picture with each phrase you want to memorize, making remembering that phrase easier. Studies have shown that combining words and pictures can be an effective way to remember things. Try it next time you're studying for an exam.

11.   Paying more attention to your surroundings and interactions with others makes it easier to remember names, facts and ideas. Ask questions about things you need to remember, for instance the spelling of a new name you hear. For instance, "Is Tracy spelled with a Y or I?" Make a comment or compliment about their name to further prime your memory with this fact. Sneak your memory tricks into conversations with others, and you will not have any issue recalling the information at a later point.

12.   Try learning a new language. Learning a new language can really help to keep your mind and memory in shape. It has also been proven to delay brain deterioration and dementia. Just immersing

yourself in the language will do. There is no need to become a fluent speaker of it.

13.   If you have trouble remembering things, don't be afraid to take notes, make lists or use a day planner to keep track of your schedule. These helpful tools can take some of the stress out of trying to remember everything on your own. Once you have lowered your stress levels by writing everything down, you may even find that your memory improves, since too much stress can inhibit memory.

14.   When it comes to memory a lot of times people find themselves having trouble remembering "boring" information such as phone numbers or addresses. The best way to make this information part of your long term memory is to store it in your mind in a way that is easy for it to retrieve later on, this means attaching an emotional connection to it so that your brain saves it in more than one area.

15.   If you are concerned about memory loss, organize your home and your life. You will not be able to remember information and events if things are messy and disorganized. Make to-do lists and use a planner. It is also crucial to keep important items, like your keys and checkbook, in the same place.

16.   Forgetting some things is natural. There is no possible way to retain every piece of information and recall it on demand. However, following the tips in this article will help you to become much more adept at remembering and retaining information you have learned. Follow the tips above for great memory.

17.   Try writing things down to make it easier to remember. Not only does this circulate blood to the part of the brain responsible for memory function, but it also exercises it. Students have been acing exams for years by taking notes, and you too can apply this technique to recall information. Just keep a diary, take thorough notes or even keep things cataloged in your PC's Word program.

18.   Keep a diary or calendar for appointments. This is extremely helpful in remembering important dates or events. Be consistent with it and keep it in the same place all the time. You should look at it every day to update it and to make sure there isn't anything you are forgetting.

19.   It is important that you take steps to keep your memory in shape throughout the years. Diet is crical in this regard. It has been shown that getting enough folic acid in your diet can help fight

memory loss. Foods rich in folic acid include many beans and legumes, leafy greens, fortified bread and cereals, citrus juices and more.

20. Most of us live in routines. Our lives are centered around having the same routine each day or each week. If we stray from that routine it can keep us from being able to remember things. Your routine is what is holding back your memory. Change how you do things each day to force your brain to develop new ways of remembering and sorting information.

21. To successfully remember information, you need to give it your complete and undivided attention. For information to move out of your short-term memory and into your long-term memory, you need to be carefully attending to it. Be sure that you read and study in a quiet place without any other distractions.

22. Getting more of your senses involved will greatly aid you in remembering! Studies suggest speaking and hearing something will reinforce your memory of it so try reading things out loud to yourself if it is important for you to remember or as a general exercise for your memory. You will see the information, say it and hear it thereby tripling your sensory exposure to it!

23.   Make your memorization easier by using mnemonic devices. The easiest one is to associate a visual image with the word or name you need to remember. Life like, vivid images linked to hard to memorize or understand concepts can help to speed up the learning process significantly. Think of images from your everyday life to make the process easier and faster.

24.   A well-nourished brain will definitely perform better in terms of memory. Eat lots of vegetables, fruits, and whole grains. Also, drink a lot of water. You should drink up to 8 glasses daily. Other ways to improve your diet is to limit the amount of saturated fat, but eat fish or supplements for omega-3 fatty acids (which improves brain function and fights against Alzheimer's).

25.   One tip for helping to remember things is to associate words and phrases with images. For example, let's say you have to do something at three o'clock. It's difficult to remember just three, but if you associate the memory with the three little pigs, you're more likely to remember what time it was that you had something to do.

26.   Draw a picture! If you are having trouble remembering something - try doodling! Drawing

relaxes your mind, opens it up. It doesn't matter if you are a terrible artist. Just scribbling on a piece of scrap paper will do. Your thoughts will feel more organized and memories will come to you much easier.

27.   Things are easier to remember if they have a special meaning to you. Think about why you need to memorize the information. For example, if you are going shopping, ask yourself why. It could be for your child's birthday and thinking about that, will help you remember what you need to buy.

28.   If you have forgotten something important that you need to remember, close your eyes and take a deep breath. Try breathing exercises by holding your breath in for a few seconds and releasing it. After doing this a few times, go back to trying to remember what you have forgotten.

29.   Try working on learning a new skill if your brain feels unfocused and your memory is lacking. New skills use new parts of the brain and force you to expand your ways of thinking. Learn to juggle, build something, try martial arts, or take a cooking class to broaden your brain's abilities.

30.   If you are trying to remember things, put your focus solely onto what you are learning. Long-term

memory plays an important role in remembering things. Distractions interfere with the process of storing information in long-term memory.

31.   Paying true attention can go a long way when you try and recall things. When you meet someone for the first time, try to imagine how to spell their name in your mind or ask them about the spelling. You can simply ask how their name is spelled. Make a comment or compliment about their name to further prime your memory with this fact. Use new names right away, and you should be able to remember them later.

32.   If you have something you'd like to commit to memory, pick your favorite tune and set to words you'd like to recall to it. This can be effective, you can see it from kids who learn the alphabet song. Melodies are repetitive, and your brain holds on to them easily. So, sing your next thought and see how easily you recall it.

33.   Avoid cramming all your material into one short study session. Studies show that information is better retained, if you take some time to learn it. You can do this by scheduling short study sessions in the days and weeks, prior to an exam. Cramming everything into one sitting will only prove to be counter productive.

34.   One fun way to improve your memory is by playing games designed to challenge your brain. It is important to exercise your brain, just like it's important to exercise your body. Regular exercise of your brain helps it to become stronger, and will improve your memory, focus and concentration skills. Good games include things like crossword puzzles, chess and word challenges. Scrabble is a good, fun daily challenge.

35.   One thing that has been proven to help maintain your memory and brain function over time, is socialization. Having a strong social group and lots of interaction and conversation with family and friends will help to keep your memory flowing freely both now and as you age too.

36.   It is easier to remember information if you organize the material into related groups, before trying to commit it to memory. Making an outline is another good way to organize the material to be studied. This is similar to how your brain organizes information and will make recall simpler.

37.   When a person is sleep deprived, his brain struggles to be fully functioning. Simple things like problem-solving, creative thinking and remembering, suddenly become difficult. Getting a

full night's rest each and every night will maintain your brain's ability to function at capacity. Enough sleep also increases your memory since the most important memory enhancing activities occur while you are in your deepest sleep.

38.   If you find yourself having difficulty recalling information, take a deep breath and relax. Sometimes all you need is a bit more time to allow your memory to retrieve the information. Feeling pressed for time can result in stress that inhibits the recall process. Remember that the older you are, the longer it takes to retrieve information from the memory.

39.   The health of your body has a direct impact on the health of your memory. The brain is an organ just like your heart or lungs. Activities that improve your physical well being will ensure that it functions at the highest level possible. Take care of yourself, rest, eat a healthy diet and exercise.

40.   To try to remember more things. You may want to create a catchy song. People find that putting important information into a song helps their memory. Try to find words that rhyme, and do not put anything too complicated into the song, as that could just end up confusing you more.

41.   Try to stay away from pills that promise to help improve your memory. Most of the time, these pills are not effective and could cause you physical problems. Instead, you may want to look into supplements like Niacin, Thiamine, and Vitamin B-6. They all help to improve the part of the brain that deals with memory.

42.   If you are trying to remember some body of information, one of the best techniques for doing so is to try to teach it to someone else. Teaching concepts to another person actually improves understanding and recall for both the student and the teacher. Even something as simple as reading out loud to someone else can help too.

43.   Loss of memory is easily one of the worst things that can happen to an aging mind. Prescription medication may be the most effective course of treatment if memory impairment is caused by an actual medical condition--dementia or Alzheimer's, for instance.

44.   Knowing what type of learner you are will enable you to reinforce your memory! If you know that you are a visual learner, for example, then keep a small notebook with you at all times to write down the information you need to remember, or if you are an auditory learner, use a small recorder.

These small aids will be a big help when you need to call on your memory later!

45.   If memory loss or simply poor memory is your problem perhaps an Omega 3 deficiency is at the heart of the problem. Try taking an Omega 3 supplement, or a medication like Lovaza to help with this. Researchers have discovered in Britain that children who were supplemented with Omega 2 were more focused and had better memory.

46.   A good tip to help improve your memory is to be more social. Studies have shown that our brains respond much better to socializing than if we were alone. People who socialize regularly will enjoy the benefit of a slower memory decline. Try being more social to improve your memory.

47.   If you feel that your memory is suffering, try to reduce stress, anger, and especially depression in your life. One of the primary symptoms of depression is actually an inability to concentrate, which makes it extremely difficult to acquire and retain memories. See a professional if you think this could apply to you.

48.   The next time your memory fails to help you remember where you placed something, be sure to jog your memory. Try to remember where you last

placed something and how long ago it was. From now on, try to keep your items in the same place so you do not forget where they are.

49.   When you need to memorize something quickly you need to have intense focus. Get rid of all distractions such as outside noises, email and cell phones and find a quiet, peaceful place. Finding an uncluttered place is helpful because you need your mind to help you concentrate and not to focus on the clutter.

50.   Pay careful attention to what you want to remember to ensure the information is retained in your long-term memory. Distractions, such as music and television, prevent you from paying the required amount of attention to the material. Failure to concentrate will result in the information being lost and not committed to memory.

51.   A useful strategy when tasked with the memory of new information is to restructure and reorganize the information. The simplest way to do this is to take the information and create a summary outline in a notebook or on your computer. This works for two reasons. It is easier to remember something that you have worked with, and the process also naturally reorders the information in a way that is easier for you to remember.

52.   It is important that you stop drinking sugary drinks, like soda, when you are trying to improve your memory. Believe it or not, sugary drinks increase your blood glucose level, which in turn, deteriorates your brain function and memory. Instead, try to drink at least 8 glasses of water a day.

53.   After you learn something new, teach it to another person. When you teach it, it forces your brain to manipulate the information in another way in order for you to articulate it. This manipulation of information strengthens that part of your memory, and it is an effective way in committing the new information into your brain.

54.   If you constantly have trouble remembering certain things, find ways to eliminate the problem once and for all. For instance, if you can never remember where you placed your car keys, put a peg by your front door where you can hang your keys the minute you enter your house. Make a list of the items you most frequently forget and then figure out a simple way to remember each of the items on your list.

55.   When trying to commit information into your long-term memory, make sure you are in a location with zero distractions. It takes real attention to

move information from short-term to long-term memory, and a distracting environment can make the task nearly impossible. Steer clear of areas where there are televisions, radios, crowds or lots of visual stimuli.

56.   It is important that you keep a daily routine if you want to improve your memory. By doing things at different times of the day, you may forget certain obligations. Try to stick with one routine for the weekdays when you are at work and one routine for weekends when you are home.

57.   Pay attention when you want to memorize something. Clear your mind completely and focus on the subject and avoid outside distractions such as noises and images. Persons with focusing difficulties should find a silent, remote location to improve focusing and speeding up the memorization process. Use pleasant music to enhance your focusing.

58.   As if you needed another excuse to exercise, physical activity enhances the effects of helpful chemicals within the brain and actually protects brain cells! Exercise is one potent weapon in improving your memory or maintaining more of it, as you get older. So keep active, keep moving and keep more in memory!

59.   Use mnemonic devices to help you remember things. Mnemonic devices are sets of clues that helps by associating things that are usually hard to remember with things that are easier to remember. An example is using an acronym, rhymes, visual images, or even associating a funny story to whatever you want to memorize.

60.   If you are a student studying for a test, it is important not to over study. Of course it is natural to want to remember information on the test, but by studying too much you are actually overworking your brain cells, which in turn could cause you to not remember anything.

61.   Visualizing information in your brain works well for many people. You only have to remember a small piece of information at a time, rather than a large amount at once. An example of this is a phone number. It is much easier to recall 888-990-8765 than it is to remember 8889908765.

62.   Use all of your senses to help your memorize. All of your senses use different portions of your brain, so you will not have to work as hard to recall the information. Visualize the item, smell it (if you can) and taste it (if it is food). The more effort you

put into visualizing the object, the easier it will be to recall.

63.   Get sufficient sleep. Getting enough sleep is important to keeping your memory sharp. When you are asleep, your brain disposes of unnecessary memories and forms more storage for new information. If you fail to get enough sleep, your brain doesn't have enough time to recharge. You will find you have trouble focusing.

64.   If you are studying complicated information that you know nothing about, try to link it to a topic that you are very familiar with. You will be able to recall the unfamiliar material much better if you are able to associate it with something that is easy for you to understand.

65.   Use a visualization technique to help you remember information. Most people can recall study material better if they are able to associate it with a picture. You may be able to link a chart or picture in your study book to your information or you can make your own image by drawing graphs or figures.

66.   To help you remember what you have to do for the day, set reminders. For instance, if you have to pay bills set an object on top them that's out of

place. Seeing the out of place object will be the reminder you need to pay your bills.

67.   Your memory is only as good as the effort you put in to maintaining it. If you believe that you have are eventually going to have a poor memory no matter what, then it can become a self-fulfilling prophesy. Give yourself positive reinforcement when you do recall something correctly and forgive yourself if you make a mistake. Your memory should begin to improve in no time. Of course, you also need to be eating and sleeping well - and go easy on the alcohol!

68.   When learning a new concept, teaching someone else the concept has been proven to be an effective way to improve your memory. The reason for this is that when you teach someone else the concept, you must first have an understanding of it and then be able to phrase it yourself. It is significantly more effective than simply trying to remember a concept word for word.

69.   Keep your memory fresh by removing stress. When you are feeling stressed about something it can be harder to pull up memorized data. Find ways to relax yourself before you have to rely on your memory for a task. Meditate for a bit on relaxing

thoughts that will allow your brain to process the information you need to access.

70. Don't skip on the sleep if you want to improve your memory. It is when we sleep that our brains really go to work. During deep sleep our brains are incredibly active in processing information and trying to understand problems. Skimping on your sleep will start having an almost immediate effect on your memory.

71. Try to visualize what you are trying to remember. When you see a mental picture of what you want to learn, you can recall it better. Visualize things like images, charts, or special aspects of the material that you are reading. When you remember those characteristics, you can recall the material more effectively.

72. Being the proverbial social butterfly can actually help to strengthen your memory. Social interactions improve your state of mind, which has the effect of making you more alert and receptive to learning things. Depressed people don't properly stimulate their mind, meaning their brain won't get the necessary exercise it needs. Exciting and interesting conversations with friends and family helps stimulate and exercise your brain, which then helps you improve your memory.

73.   Be sure to visit a dentist and take good care of your teeth if you want to have a good memory. Tooth and gum disease have been known to clog your carotid arteries, which in turn decreases oxygen to the brain. Without enough oxygen, the brain cannot process and keep information.

74.   To better commit names to memory, repeat a person's name after an introduction, and try to come up with something about the person that might help you remember his or her name. If you meet a Bob who mentions that he enjoys fishing, you might associate his name with a bobber like those used on a fishing line, for instance.

75.   When trying to commit information into your long-term memory, make sure you are in a location with zero distractions. It takes real attention to move information from short-term to long-term memory, and a distracting environment can make the task nearly impossible. Steer clear of areas where there are televisions, radios, crowds or lots of visual stimuli.

76.   Get plenty of sleep. Studies indicate that your short-term memory can be negatively affected by a lack of sleep. A lack of concentration will lead to a

great deal of difficulty in turning present happenings into permanent memories.

77.   If someone you know is suffering from Dementia, Alzheimer's Disease, or another illness that effects their memory, try showing them pleasant pictures from the past. By looking at pleasant memories, the memory of these patients may improve. Be sure not to bring up unpleasant memories as this could cause them a setback.

78.   Add aromatherapy to your life if you want to improve your memory. This works because these aromas help to relax you, which in turn, helps your memory improve. Also, if you are not sensitive to the smells, you may want to try adding candles throughout your home as they will relax you too.

79.   Sleep is vital to maintaining mental clarity and memory. By avoiding sleep, you make your senses and mind foggier, hurting your ability to focus and piece together information. In addition, during sleep, your brain forges pathways that lead to memory. Getting good sleep (and a good amount of it) will improve your memory.

80.   Paying attention to what you are doing will help your memory. When studying or memorizing something, avoid distractions. Find an environment

you are comfortable in. Learn how to focus on something, and if you can, find material that interest you. Focusing on something that interest you should be relatively easy.

81.   Remembering and matching names with faces can be very difficult. Focus on the person's face or a specific feature of their face; then try recalling an anecdote about them. With time and practice people's names will spring to mind more readily.

82.   In order to remember information, one key idea is to rehearse the information out loud. By repeating the information over and over to yourself or others you will maximize your chances for being able to recall it later. Even developing flash cards will be helpful to help you remember the data.

83.   Try your best to stay in the moment when you are learning. If you are distracted by the past or the future, you'll never absorb what you want to learn right now. If you're feeling overwhelmed by other events in your life, take a break and come back to learning later.

84.   If you have noticed that your memory isn't what it used to be, maybe you aren't getting enough sleep. You need to be sleeping seven to eight hours each night in order to improve your memory. During

your sleep cycle, your brain processes all new information to create these memories for you so you have them to recall later.

85.   Keep a running list of the things you want to accomplish each day. As you finish one item, cross it off and move on to the next. Simultaneously, keep adding items at the bottom of the list as they arise. In this way you will never forget what you need to do next.

86.   When trying to remember any type of information the key is repetition. The more something is repeated in your mind the more likely you are to keep it in your long term memory. For example, if you meet someone new, repeat their name in your head at least three times while looking at them.

87.   A good way to help you remember things is to keep repeating them outloud. Eventually, this information is going to be embedded into your head if you keep hearing it over and over again. For instance, if you have to clean your room on Saturday, keep saying so outloud.

88.   The easiest way to improve your memory is to get a good night's sleep! Sometimes our busy schedules make it seem like cutting out a few hours

of sleep is the only way to be productive, but your brain needs rest to function at its best. Sleeping is also when your brain processes and stores your memories from that day.

89.   Although it is a fact that many people do not know, chewing gum can improve your memory. Medical professionals have found that the motion of chewing gum slightly increases your heart rate. Even the slightest increase in heart rate can help supply more oxygen to the brain, thus improving memory.

90.   A well-nourished brain will definitely perform better in terms of memory. Eat lots of vegetables, fruits, and whole grains. Also, drink a lot of water. You should drink up to 8 glasses daily. Other ways to improve your diet is to limit the amount of saturated fat, but eat fish or supplements for omega-3 fatty acids (which improves brain function and fights against Alzheimer's).

91.   A memory technique that works for many people is the listen, write and read method. Basically what this entails is really listening to what is being said. While listening, make notes about the material that is being shared. At a later time, read the notes again. With this technique, you are actually

reviewing the information three times which aids in cementing the information in your memory.

92.   Carefully focus on what you are trying to memorize. This is especially important when you are studying. Never try to multitask. Turn off the television, turn off the radio. Just focus on what you need to memorize and the knowledge you need to retain. Many things can distract you without you even realizing it.

93.   If you are having trouble remembering what someone has told you, try to rephrase what is being said. As long as you are keeping the original meaning alive, it can be very helpful for remembering the information. Memorization is difficult if people do not have a grasp of what the words mean.

94.   You need to make sure you focus on the information that you are trying to remember. If you are trying to remember a shopping list, try visualizing the items or write them down to jog your memory. Take your time to repeat information after you hear it so it has a chance of sticking with you.

95.   Recognize that your memories might be biased. How you perceive the world will always be from

your point of view. Because of that, your memories of things will always be ever so slightly biased in your favor. It is important to recognize and compensate for this. To recall an event correctly, try recalling it from an objective point of view.

96.   If you have a visual type of memory, use pictures, drawings and graphs to remember information. If this visual material is not a part of what you need to learn, you can easily create it yourself. Make sure you create clear pictures you will be able to understand later when you go over your information again.

97.   If you want to boost your memory, start by finding ways to reduce stress. When you experience stress, your body release cortisol. This hormone reduces the ability of your brain to recall old memories or store new ones. By reducing your stress levels, you can reduce the amount of cortisol in your system and in turn improve your memory.

98.   A key component to memory is to give yourself less to memorize. Instead of having to remember where you put your keys, always put your keys in the same place so that you only have to memorize where you always put your keys, instead of where you put them this one time. This same principle applies to memorizing many things.

99.	Using acronyms is a great way to help you remember things. Acronyms are formed by using the first letter from a group of words to make a new word. This comes in handy when you are learning something ins a specific order. For example, if you are trying to remember the colors of the rainbow, you can remember ROY G BIV (red, orange, yellow, green, blue, indigo and violet).

100.	A great way for you to improve your overall memory is to make sure that you're always focusing your attentions on whatever you're studying at the time. The goal here is knowledge retention. A failure to focus fully on the subject at hand means the information may not be retained properly.

101.	A great tip for improving your memory is to deliberately increase your intake of fish oil, which is known to boost concentration and recall. By seeking foods high in Omega-3 acids or taking fish oil supplements, it is possible to experience noticeable improvement in your ability to remember important things.

102.	If you have a hard time remembering to do important things, you may want to leave yourself a voice message. Looking at your phone and seeing that you have a message will help to remind you that you have something important thing to do. Text messaging is another convenient reminder technique.

103.   When trying to commit something to memory, it is important to maintain low stress levels. This is because stress and anxiety can quickly cause you to lose your concentration. Concentration is necessary for acquiring new information. A good solution is to listen to soothing music. Music can help to keep your stress levels down, by keeping your mind off of the things that cause you to be anxious.

104.   To keep your memory in tip-top shape, practice using it regularly. If you don't use your memory, it will slowly become weaker and weaker over time. The best way to keep it in shape is by regularly challenging it in your day to day life. This can be something as simple as doing a crossword puzzle or as complex as trying to memorize the names of all of the members of the arachnid family. Just find fun ways to test and challenge your memory each and every day.

105.   To help improve how quickly something is stored in your memory, take the time to bucket the information first. Act like an information architect and organize the information you are try to commit to memory based off of similarities. Once they are

bucketed, attack them as a group. You will then find they are easier to memorize!

106.   A great technique to help you memorize new material is to read the information out loud. Research has shown that this simple act significantly improves the memory of this material. Research has also divulged that teaching a new concept to others will also increase understanding and recall of the information.

107.   Improve memory with mnemonics. Use an acronym to remember lists of related things. For example, 'Homes' is used to remember the names of the Great Lakes: Huron, Ontario, Michigan, Erie and Superior. The first letter of the words in a sentence can represent a list of letters that you have to remember. For example, "Every good boy does fine" can be used to memorize the notes on the lines of a treble clef: E,G,B,D and F.

108.   If you have trouble remembering words or names, try repeating them out loud. For instance, if you are introduced to a new person, repeat their name back to them by saying something like "Nice to meet you, Susan." This simple tip will help to cement the word or name in your mind, so you can easily recall it when you need to.

109.   Before you make a commitment to improve your memory, be sure you are all ready to do so and keep an open mind. Some people's memories will not improve because they are not willing to try certain techniques given to them. Tell yourself that with enough hard work, your memory will work fine in no time!

110.   Put more effort into maintaining existing relationships as well as into building new ones to help fortify your brain against memory loss. Studies have shown that spending time with your loved ones, even if it is for a few hours a week, is healthy for the part of your brain that holds memories.

111.   One way to improve your memory is by adding meditation to your daily routine. Meditating helps to relax your mind and body, which in turn can make it easier for your brain to recall memories. Set aside a specific time each day when you know you won't be interrupted to close your eyes and meditate for as long as you would like.

112.   When trying to memorize a large bit of information or a number which is long, you can retain the information by learning it in chunks. Take the information and group it into small segments that you are able to easily retain. When you have the

small segments memorized, add the groups together two at a time until you have remembered it all.

113.   A good approach to studying is to separate the categories you want to master into related groups. This is found to be much better than trying to learn things in a random, haphazard order. Scientists have indicated that this type of mental organization facilitates better recollection down the road.

114.   If you are concerned about memory loss, organize your home and your life. You will not be able to remember information and events if things are messy and disorganized. Make to-do lists and use a planner. It is also crucial to keep important items, like your keys and checkbook, in the same place.

115.   To help you easily remember and recall information, it helps to organize information. Group the information by rational relationships. For example, if you are trying to remember if you want to learn all the American presidents, you can organize their names by political party, their platform or the state they are from. Doing it this way, can make it easier to recall them if you organize them in one of these ways.

116.   If you are having memory problems, try taking fish oil. Recent studies have shown a link between problems with concentration and memory and a deficiency in Omega-3 fatty acids. One of the best Omega-3 sources is fish oil. You can either take the oil in the liquid form by the spoonful, or opt for fish oil pills instead.

117.   If so, allow yourself a brief break, but no longer than 15 minutes, during every hour and use that time to rest your mind. This will get your brain in the right state to more readily absorb new information.

118.   The health of your body has a direct impact on the health of your memory. The brain is an organ just like your heart or lungs. Activities that improve your physical well being will ensure that it functions at the highest level possible. Take care of yourself, rest, eat a healthy diet and exercise.

119.   When learning a new concept, teaching someone else the concept has been proven to be an effective way to improve your memory. The reason for this is that when you teach someone else the concept, you must first have an understanding of it and then be able to phrase it yourself. It is significantly more effective than simply trying to remember a concept word for word.

120.   A good way to help you remember things is to keep repeating them outloud. Eventually, this information is going to be embedded into your head if you keep hearing it over and over again. For instance, if you have to clean your room on Saturday, keep saying so outloud.

121.   Don't skip on the sleep if you want to improve your memory. It is when we sleep that our brains really go to work. During deep sleep our brains are incredibly active in processing information and trying to understand problems. Skimping on your sleep will start having an almost immediate effect on your memory.

122.   It is important that you get good quality sleep. You may not know it, but the amount of sleep that you get can play a large role in your ability to retain information. If you have a tired mind, you'll have a tough time remembering things. Just get additional sleep at night and watch your memory improve.

123.   When trying to remember something, having patience with yourself will help you greatly! The harder you try to think of something, the more stressed you become, and of course, the more stressed you become the more difficult it is to remember anything! Take a deep breath, relax, and

try to clear your mind and before you know it what ever you were trying so hard to recall will pop right up in your mind!

124.   Improve memory with mnemonics. Use an acronym to remember lists of related things. For example, 'Homes' is used to remember the names of the Great Lakes: Huron, Ontario, Michigan, Erie and Superior. The first letter of the words in a sentence can represent a list of letters that you have to remember. For example, "Every good boy does fine" can be used to memorize the notes on the lines of a treble clef: E,G,B,D and F.

125.   When learning new information, try forming a visual image of it in your mind. When your brain is forced to come up with a picture to go along with the information, it has to analyze it more carefully that it otherwise would have. This attention to detail can help cement it in your mind. Not only that, but you can use the mental image that you formed to help you recall the information at a later date.

126.   A good tip to help improve your memory is to be more social. Studies have shown that our brains respond much better to socializing than if we were alone. People who socialize regularly will enjoy the benefit of a slower memory decline. Try being more social to improve your memory.

127.   A great tip that can help you improve your memory is to make sure you're getting enough healthy fats in your diet that contain omega-3's. These healthy fats are great because they support brain health. You can find omega-3's in salmon, flaxseed, or you can just take a fish oil supplement.

128.   Say things out loud. Anytime you learn a new name, repeat it verbally. By repeating these things out loud for you to hear will ensure you remember this information for future use. Multiple repetitions are a good idea any place where you are alone, unless you're not shy about doing this in the company of others.

129.   A good way to remember names and improve memory is to use pictures to associate with the names. If the persons name is Bob Frost, try to remember them covered in frost. If the persons name is Gemma Hand, try to picture them standing and applauding giving someone standing ovation or giving them a hand moving.

130.   When trying to commit an item such as study materials to memory, it is best that you focus on these in an environment which is free from distractions such as television or music. Items can only move from the short term memory into the

long term memory if you actively pay attention to the topic on hand.

131.   When trying to memorize a large bit of information or a number which is long, you can retain the information by learning it in chunks. Take the information and group it into small segments that you are able to easily retain. When you have the small segments memorized, add the groups together two at a time until you have remembered it all.

132.   Try taking a brain boosting vitamin. Certain nutrients have been shown to affect our memory and brain function overall. Ginko Biloba and others are quite often considered to be the best at it. Take a vitamin that is geared towards memory retention or look for ways to incorporate foods rich in these nutrients into your diet.

133.   Keep a running list of the things you want to accomplish each day. As you finish one item, cross it off and move on to the next. Simultaneously, keep adding items at the bottom of the list as they arise. In this way you will never forget what you need to do next.

134.   Take advantage of social networking sites to remember birthdays. Take the time to invite all your friends to join you on your social networking site,

and be sure to ask them when their birthdays are and enter this information in the birthday reminder program provided so that you will always be notified in advance.

135. Try to stay away from pills that promise to help improve your memory. Most of the time, these pills are not effective and could cause you physical problems. Instead, you may want to look into supplements like Niacin, Thiamine, and Vitamin B-6. They all help to improve the part of the brain that deals with memory.

136. To help improve your memory and overall brain function, try to eat a healthy diet. Studies have shown that eating certain foods can help improve a person's memory. Spinach and many fruits, including blueberries, help memory function. Omega-3 fatty acids is also beneficial when trying to improve memory.

137. It is important to get a sufficient amount of sleep if you are trying to improve your memory. Medical studies have shown that getting enough sleep every night can improve both short and long term memory. Your brain cannot absorb new information when your body has not gotten a lot of sleep.

138.   It is important that you take steps to keep your memory in shape throughout the years. Diet is crical in this regard. It has been shown that getting enough folic acid in your diet can help fight memory loss. Foods rich in folic acid include many beans and legumes, leafy greens, fortified bread and cereals, citrus juices and more.

139.   After you learn something new, teach it to another person. When you teach it, it forces your brain to manipulate the information in another way in order for you to articulate it. This manipulation of information strengthens that part of your memory, and it is an effective way in committing the new information into your brain.

140.   To successfully remember information, you need to give it your complete and undivided attention. For information to move out of your short-term memory and into your long-term memory, you need to be carefully attending to it. Be sure that you read and study in a quiet place without any other distractions.

141.   One way to improve memory is to employ mnemonics. For example, when musicians learn the treble clef they learn "every good boy deserves fudge." This simplifies the learning of the notes on the lines of the treble clef without overly burdening

the memory. Simple mnemonic device make learning new things much easier.

142.   Teaching others is a great way to keep your memory sharp. Telling the story of when you showed your grandchild how to swim to others, will help you remember the event more clearly. This way, you can, and will, reinforce this in your mind, and make it far more difficult to forget.

143.   If you feel that your memory is suffering, try to reduce stress, anger, and especially depression in your life. One of the primary symptoms of depression is actually an inability to concentrate, which makes it extremely difficult to acquire and retain memories. See a professional if you think this could apply to you.

144.   If you find that you are losing things as soon as you set them down, try dedicating a spot to them. Make sure that you are putting your keys in the same spot every day. Make a spot for your glasses or the book you are reading. If you make a habit of putting everything in its place, forgetting where they are won't be a problem.

145.   Did you know that, even late in life, you can grow new brain cells within the memory center of your brain? Recent research has revealed that high-

level aerobic exercise, such as running and bicycling, actually stimulates the growth of new brain neurons within the brain's hippocampus. If you want to have a better memory, adding more aerobic exercise to your daily activities will help.

146.   A great way to improve memory and brain elasticity is to read a large variety of books. Read novels from all eras and places as well as histories, self help books, nonfiction books, and anything else you can find. The different types of information you take in give your brain a workout.

147.   Mnemonic devices can be a powerful strategy to use when you want to remember something important. This technique involves pairing something you have to remember with something that you know very well. They usually involve jokes, songs or rhymes and are an enjoyable method to improve memory. They can even remove irritation and frustration from studying.

148.   Pay careful attention to what you want to remember to ensure the information is retained in your long-term memory. Distractions, such as music and television, prevent you from paying the required amount of attention to the material. Failure to concentrate will result in the information being lost and not committed to memory.

149.   It is easier to remember information if you organize the material into related groups, before trying to commit it to memory. Making an outline is another good way to organize the material to be studied. This is similar to how your brain organizes information and will make recall simpler.

150.   If you need to remember a complicated piece of information, use the mnemonics technique. This is a way of associating the information with something that is common and familiar. When you make that association, you can think of the common item, and it will trigger your memory of the more complicated piece of information.

151.   A useful memory tip for anyone needing to recall particular types of information, is to work on minimizing distractions in your surroundings. Competing stimuli can actually impede recollection and prevent easy access to stored information. By seeking peace and quiet, it will be easier to retrieve the desired data from your mind.

152.   Help protect your memory for years to come by making sure you are getting plenty of vitamin B-12 in your diet. Studies have linked low levels of B-12 to dementia and poor cognitive function. Food sources rich in B-12 include liver, eggs, fish, poultry,

meat and milk products. If you don't eat a lot of meat, you may need to take a daily B-12 supplement to help prevent deficiency.

153.   To improve absorbing and remembering things, try using Mnemonics tricks. These are mind games that are often used by children in school when trying to learn things. For example, people use "I before E, except after C" to remember that in the English language, the letter "I" always goes before "E" in words, except after the letter "C".

154.   Believing you have a poor memory is a self-fulfilling prophecy! If you are constantly telling yourself and other people that you have a bad memory, then that is exactly what you will have! As with anything, keeping a positive attitude will improve the situation so stop reminding yourself that you are forgetful and as your outlook improves, so will your memory!

155.   If you are trying to remember a large list of items, try placing them in categories. For instance, if you are headed to the grocery store and have a number of items that you want to get while are there, mentally group them into categories such as meat, dairy, produce and grains. Breaking down big lists into smaller subcategories makes them far easier to remember.

156.   Use memorization techniques and drills to continually challenge your mind to retain more information. Using these techniques and drills, allows you to improve your memory, while also remembering vital information, like telephone numbers and definitions. The list of data you can use for these techniques is limitless and can also, help you in your daily activities.

157.   If you are finding your memory is lacking it may be because of a lack of sleep. As such try getting more rest. Scientists believe that when we are asleep it is when our brain sorts through the events of our lives and files them away, like a librarian and a filing cabinet. They also believe this is why we dream.

158.   A great tip that can help you improve your memory is to make sure you're getting enough healthy fats in your diet that contain omega-3's. These healthy fats are great because they support brain health. You can find omega-3's in salmon, flaxseed, or you can just take a fish oil supplement.

159.   A great way to help you improve your memory is to start taking alternative driving routes. Taking different routes will keep your mind active by keeping you guessing and alert. Keeping your mind

active like this can go a long way in improving your ability to remember things.

160.   To improve your memory, make sure you are getting enough exercise, but especially of the aerobic variety. Recent research indicates that concentrated aerobic exercise activities actually encourage new cell growth in the brain's memory center. Try to do aerobic exercises such as biking and running in order to get the maximum benefit.

161.   You can feel healthier, relieve anxiety, and improve your brain and memory by practicing meditation techniques. Meditating is as simple as getting comfortable and then focusing all of your energy and attention on controlling your breathing pattern. Work at meditating for thirty minutes a day at the minimum to help keep your brain in shape.

162.   Classical music may improve your memory. Music which causes you to relax your mind and body might also help improve your memory. An excellent time for playing this type of music is when taking a hot, relaxing bath. In this bath, consider having some candles burning.

163.   A way to improve brain function and memory is to mix things up in your daily routine. Humans get attached to routines and hobbies and doing the

same thing repeatedly, but the more something is ingrained in us, the less effort it takes the brain to carry out. Try little new things like going to the store a different way or opening all doors with the wrong hand to keep your brain on its toes.

164.   Spend more time on the information you are having trouble remembering. Go over what you need to remember a couple of times and see what was easy to remember for you. Pay more attention to what seems difficult. Rephrase this content in a way that makes it easy to remember.

165.   Pay careful attention to what you want to remember to ensure the information is retained in your long-term memory. Distractions, such as music and television, prevent you from paying the required amount of attention to the material. Failure to concentrate will result in the information being lost and not committed to memory.

166.   If you have noticed that your memory isn't what it used to be, maybe you aren't getting enough sleep. You need to be sleeping seven to eight hours each night in order to improve your memory. During your sleep cycle, your brain processes all new information to create these memories for you so you have them to recall later.

167.   Your brain is like a muscle; you have to work it out to keep your memory sharp. You can improve brain function and potentially stop your brain from degenerating with age if you challenge your brain with puzzles.

168.   To improve your memory, try a glass or two of wine. You may be surprised to know that wine in moderation can help improve your memory. Red wines are the highest in resveratrol, a chemical that increases your brain power and may even prevent Alzheimer's disease. Just don't drink too much or it may hurt your memory instead of helping it!

169.   Exercise regularly as it can improve your memory functions and health. Physical exercises improve your physical look and they also increase the oxygen flow to the brain. A physically well kept body is less prone to catch memory loss causing illnesses and increases the useful brain chemicals' presence in the blood.

170.   Eat a healthy diet to keep your memory strong. Your brain needs the proper nutrients to keep the brain cells healthy. A healthy diet includes keeping your body properly hydrated and reducing alcohol intake. Alcohol confuses the mind; too much of it adversely affects your memory. Your diet should include low-sugar and low-fat foods.

171.   A slipping memory is a tragic event for a mind advancing in age. For those suffering from serious memory loss, there are a number of medical treatments available today including prescription medications.

172.   If you are having issues with remembering things, you may want to try relaxing techniques like yoga or meditation. When your body is relaxed, so is your mind which allows you to easily learn and remember things. Working your mind and body to hard will make memorizing things much worse.

173.   Add aromatherapy to your life if you want to improve your memory. This works because these aromas help to relax you, which in turn, helps your memory improve. Also, if you are not sensitive to the smells, you may want to try adding candles throughout your home as they will relax you too.

174.   Challenge your memory. Push yourself to remember little details. There are many games online and on video game consoles that are specifically designed to challenge your memory. Play them regularly. Get your brain in the habit of remembering things. Your memory is like a muscle. You need to exercise it.

175.   If you are a person who easily forgets things, make a mental checklist before leaving your home. Ask yourself what you usually bring with you and check to make sure that you have it. By doing this, you are reducing the risk of going somewhere without something you may really need.

176.   Try visual association to help with memory issues. The technique basically entails putting a picture with each phrase you want to memorize, making remembering that phrase easier. Studies have shown that combining words and pictures can be an effective way to remember things. Try it next time you're studying for an exam.

177.   Recognize that your memories might be biased. How you perceive the world will always be from your point of view. Because of that, your memories of things will always be ever so slightly biased in your favor. It is important to recognize and compensate for this. To recall an event correctly, try recalling it from an objective point of view.

178.   Learn how to use mnemonic devices. Mnemonic devices can be the association of a concept with a familiar object or remember acronyms or rhymes. Create your own mnemonic devices: you need to make sure they are meaningful and that you will

remember what you associated the information with later on.

179.   One of the most effective and easiest ways to remember material is by repeating it until you can easily recall it. If the information you need to remember is written down, just read it over and over until it all sinks in. It also helps to recite the information just before bed.

180.   To strengthen your recall, perform brain exercises. You can do this by practicing doing things with your less dominant hand. Try things like brushing your teeth with the 'wrong' hand. The concentration it takes will help to improve the strength of your mind. Also, memorize trivia and odd facts. This will help to enhance your memory.

181.   Have you ever put down something somewhere and then later couldn't remember where it was? In order to help your brain with memory retention try setting things down and saying aloud to yourself what you are doing, such as "I am putting the keys on the top of my dresser in my bedroom." The effort of stating the sentence aloud will help your brain to retrace that memory later when you need to find your keys.

182.   Avoid cramming all your material into one short study session. Studies show that information is better retained, if you take some time to learn it. You can do this by scheduling short study sessions in the days and weeks, prior to an exam. Cramming everything into one sitting will only prove to be counter productive.

183.   If you have noticed that your memory isn't what it used to be, maybe you aren't getting enough sleep. You need to be sleeping seven to eight hours each night in order to improve your memory. During your sleep cycle, your brain processes all new information to create these memories for you so you have them to recall later.

184.   If you really want to perform an exercise that helps you remember things, then simply write them down. Writing things out can stimulate the brain, and bring blood to critical areas that are responsible for memory. You may significantly increase your ability to remember important things by making a habit of letter writing or journaling.

185.   If you're a student trying to boost your memory for a test, the worst thing you can do is cram. Attempting to learn so much in too little time will not allow you to retain anything at all. You will only

grasp bits of pieces of the material and will not be able to properly learn what you need to.

186.   Pay attention! This is one easy way you can improve your memory. You may try to pay attention, but sometimes the mind wanders and information is not properly stored. It is important to clear your thoughts and concentrate on what is going on around you. Use any downtime in the information stream to think over some of the ideas and commit important ones to your memory.

187.   Writing by hand is a great way to help your memory. Writing with a pen or pencil engages your brain in a different way than typing on a computer. You can either copy out a speech your trying to memorize or keep track of your daily to do list by writing in a calendar. If you've written it out, you may be able to remember without even checking your list!

188.   Memory is basically the acquisition of new information, and when you have problems concentrating, it becomes vastly more difficult to acquire new information. Most problems with concentration are linked to an Omega-3 deficiency. One effective way to counter this and thereby improve your memory is through the use of fish

oils. Incorporating fish oil supplements in your diet can help your memory.

189.   Participate in regular exercise. Exercise increases oxygen to the brain and can be helpful to your memory. It also gets blood flowing to your brain more. It can also help prevent diseases that can lead to memory loss in the future. An active body leads to an active mind.

190.   If you are trying to remember a large list of items, try placing them in categories. For instance, if you are headed to the grocery store and have a number of items that you want to get while are there, mentally group them into categories such as meat, dairy, produce and grains. Breaking down big lists into smaller subcategories makes them far easier to remember.

191.   Organizing your immediate environment will make it easier for you to remember things! Keeping your keys, wallet, cell phone and other frequently used articles all together in the same place will prevent you from having to remember where they are. Since scent can improve memory, keep your favorite scented candle in this same central location! All of this will improve your memory and save you much stress and hassle.

192.   A good way to help you study is to change up your study habits and study in a brand new environment. Changing your environment refreshes your mind, and it also makes long-term memory a lot more effective. Your brain is programmed to become more alert when something new is going on, and an alert brain is better at forming memories.

193.   If you have a large amount of information to commit to memory, a good strategy is to break the information down into many separate pieces. It is much easier to remember things in parts, than to remember them as a whole. As a simple example, when trying to memorize a standard United States phone number, you can memorize it as three separate parts consisting of area code, first three digits, and last four digits, as opposed to all ten digits together.

194.   Memory loss can be a very tragic experience. Prescription medication is often used to help fight off signs of memory loss and dementia.

195.   A great tip that can help you improve your memory is to review information shortly after you've learned it. Doing this periodically will help you recall important things. What you don't want to do is cram. If you cram you won't retain as much information as you want.

196.   A great way to help you improve your memory is to start taking alternative driving routes. Taking different routes will keep your mind active by keeping you guessing and alert. Keeping your mind active like this can go a long way in improving your ability to remember things.

197.   If you are wanting to remember something new, say it! Any new material that you want to remember should be read aloud. When you read words out loud, you form a memory pathway through two of your senses, sight and hearing. This gives two paths of retrieval when you want to recall this information at a future date.

198.   Exercise your brain. Using your memory and other thought provoking functions of your brain daily, will help keep your mind and your memory sharp. Do puzzles, drive a different way to work and memorize something every day. You will see an improvement quickly and less of a decline as time moves on.

199.   Take advantage of social networking sites to remember birthdays. Take the time to invite all your friends to join you on your social networking site, and be sure to ask them when their birthdays are and enter this information in the birthday reminder

program provided so that you will always be notified in advance.

200.   If you're a student trying to boost your memory for a test, the worst thing you can do is cram. Attempting to learn so much in too little time will not allow you to retain anything at all. You will only grasp bits of pieces of the material and will not be able to properly learn what you need to.

201.   You might find mnemonic devices useful in retaining and recalling some memories. Mnemonics can be used in a similar way to how writers use shorthand. By associating a bit of information with a word or item, you can make the correlation that helps you recall it at a later time.

202.   Eat more onions to improve your memory. A few studies have isolated fisetin to be of great benefit in improving the long term memory. You can find beneficial levels of fisetin in onions, strawberries, mangos and other plants. It also is a strong antioxidant so it will deliver other benefits to your body as well.

203.   Avoid smoking cigarettes to keep your memory from being negatively affected. Studies have shown that the memory of smokers suffers more than compared to non-smokers. You probably didn't

need yet another reason to quit, but maybe this will be the one that lets you finally put down that pack.

204.   A good tip to help improve your memory is to be more social. Studies have shown that our brains respond much better to socializing than if we were alone. People who socialize regularly will enjoy the benefit of a slower memory decline. Try being more social to improve your memory.

205.   Try meditating. Meditation can help you against anxiety, depression, and stress. Studies show that regular meditators have much more activity in the the left pre-frontal cortex. This special area of the brain is associated with feelings of joy and equanimity. This also allows the brain to make more connections with brain cells, increasing memory and mental sharpness.

206.   A great tip that can help you improve your memory is to make sure you're getting enough healthy fats in your diet that contain omega-3's. These healthy fats are great because they support brain health. You can find omega-3's in salmon, flaxseed, or you can just take a fish oil supplement.

207.   Do not cram. In order to properly memorize information, you need to create study sessions instead of cramming everything into one session.

Don't try to memorize everything in one sitting. This tactic will make your mind feel overwhelmed, and you will retain very little of the actual information. Study in short sessions, and your brain can remember better.

208.   One fun way to help keep your memory sharp is to play brain games, such as puzzles and logic games. These types of games will help improve attention span, concentration, mental flexibility and memory. To keep your brain in top shape, it is recommended that you play brain games at least 15 minutes each day. According to recent research, playing brain games can even aid in the prevention of Alzheimer's Disease.

209.   Before you make a commitment to improve your memory, be sure you are all ready to do so and keep an open mind. Some people's memories will not improve because they are not willing to try certain techniques given to them. Tell yourself that with enough hard work, your memory will work fine in no time!

210.   Scent has a huge impact on memory. If you keep something that you enjoy smelling right next to where you keep things, you will have an easier time recalling where the object is. For example, if you keep a plug in air freshener right next to where

you keep you wallet when you are home, you will have no problem remembering where it is.

211.   Many people who think they have a memory problem are really suffering from a general lack of focus. There are so many things competing for our attention - family, computers, telephones, televisions and more. If you want something to register in your memory so you can recall it later, you have to first focus your attention on it so your brain knows it is important to you. Just find a quiet room that is free from distractions and give yourself the time to concentrate.

212.   Healthy sleeping can help to improve memory. If you are deprived of sleep, your brain is unable to operate at full capacity. Your problem-solving abilities, creativity and critical thinking skills are all compromised. Research has proven that sleep is critical for memory consolidation, as the key memory-enhancing activity occurs during your deepest stages of sleep.

213.   If you have trouble remembering things, don't be afraid to take notes, make lists or use a day planner to keep track of your schedule. These helpful tools can take some of the stress out of trying to remember everything on your own. Once you have lowered your stress levels by writing

everything down, you may even find that your memory improves, since too much stress can inhibit memory.

214.   Avoid cramming all your material into one short study session. Studies show that information is better retained, if you take some time to learn it. You can do this by scheduling short study sessions in the days and weeks, prior to an exam. Cramming everything into one sitting will only prove to be counter productive.

215.   To boost your memory, make sure you are getting enough sleep. Sleep deprivation can seriously impair memory, causing you to forget even the most basic things in your day to day life. If you regularly have trouble sleeping, you can try natural sleep aids such as melatonin or consider talking to your doctor about prescription sleep medication instead.

216.   If you find yourself having difficulty recalling information, take a deep breath and relax. Sometimes all you need is a bit more time to allow your memory to retrieve the information. Feeling pressed for time can result in stress that inhibits the recall process. Remember that the older you are, the longer it takes to retrieve information from the memory.

217.   Use regular study sessions over a period of time rather than a single cramming session. Studies have shown that if you study material over a course of a few days, you have a better chance of remembering it than if you cram in a single night. So instead of cramming the night before a test, establish a regular study time each night or every other night.

218.   Protecting your cells is vital to keeping your brain healthy and active. Eating foods that are rich in antioxidants like blueberries, strawberries, and other fruits and veggies will give you a leg up in taking care of your brain. These antioxidants not only keep your brain working in optimum condition, they also may help slow the aging process.

219.   When trying to memorize new information, take the time and effort to think about how this unfamiliar material relates to something that you already know and understand. By finding a relationship between new concepts and previously learned material, you will increase the likelihood of committing the new information to memory.

220.   Regularly challenging your brain can help you improve your memory. Learning new, complex tasks such as a foreign language or how to play a

musical instrument will help your brain stay active. Remember the old saying "Use it or lose it?" The same thing's true for your mind!

221.   Exercise your body - exercise your brain. By exercising regularly, you increase the amount of oxygen that gets to your brain, and reduce the risk of illnesses that can contribute to memory loss, such as heart disease and diabetes. Exercise can also increase the effects of certain chemicals that help the brain to function at its best.

222.   Visualization is a proven technique that aids in remembering critical information. When studying text, utilize charts and photographs as visual cues to help you better retain the information. You may even want to make your own graphs and charts to aid you in this memory process.

223.   A great tip that can help you improve your memory is to make sure you're getting enough sleep every night. Studies have shown that people who are sleep deprived tend to be very sluggish. All of their cognitive functions, including their memory, are compromised. Getting enough sleep is very important.

224.   It may sound silly, but one way to improve memory is to surround yourself with good friends,

and to maintain an active social life. A Harvard study suggests that those who had active and fulfilling social lives, showed rates of cognitive decline significantly lower than their less socially active peers.

225.   Eating foods rich in protein will actually help your memory as well as provide good fuel for your body! Foods like fish that have large amounts of protein are high in amino acids which aid your body in the production of neurotransmitters and these neurotransmitters are invaluable to brain performance so eat well to remember better!

226.   Reduce stress in your life to improve your memory. Unrelieved stress can cause your body to produce so much cortisol that it permanently damages your hippocampus, which is the memory center of the brain. Other stress chemicals can interfere with your ability to store information, concentrate, or recall memories from earlier.

227.   If you are a person who easily forgets things, make a mental checklist before leaving your home. Ask yourself what you usually bring with you and check to make sure that you have it. By doing this, you are reducing the risk of going somewhere without something you may really need.

228.   If you have forgotten something important that you need to remember, close your eyes and take a deep breath. Try breathing exercises by holding your breath in for a few seconds and releasing it. After doing this a few times, go back to trying to remember what you have forgotten.

229.   Spend more time on the information you are having trouble remembering. Go over what you need to remember a couple of times and see what was easy to remember for you. Pay more attention to what seems difficult. Rephrase this content in a way that makes it easy to remember.

230.   To strengthen your recall, perform brain exercises. You can do this by practicing doing things with your less dominant hand. Try things like brushing your teeth with the 'wrong' hand. The concentration it takes will help to improve the strength of your mind. Also, memorize trivia and odd facts. This will help to enhance your memory.

231.   Make sure that your diet has good sources of Omega-3 fatty acids. Most commonly found in fish, these fatty acids do a superb job of keeping your brain on its toes. Numerous studies have shown a positive benefit to the brain when the diet contains omega-3's. Try adding pink salmon, walnuts and flax seed, so you can get this essential fat.

232.   Your memory is only as good as the effort you put in to maintaining it. If you believe that you have are eventually going to have a poor memory no matter what, then it can become a self-fulfilling prophesy. Give yourself positive reinforcement when you do recall something correctly and forgive yourself if you make a mistake. Your memory should begin to improve in no time. Of course, you also need to be eating and sleeping well - and go easy on the alcohol!

233.   In order to improve your memory, try doing more aerobic exercise. Recent studies have shown that high intensity cardio workouts can actually help you grow more brain cells in your hippocampus, the portion of your brain responsible for memory. Some exercises that you may want to try include running, biking, kickboxing and swimming.

234.   If you find yourself having difficulty remembering some things, try to use acronyms or tricks called mnemonics to help you remember. An example of this is to use Roy G. Biv to remember the colors of the rainbow as red, orange, yellow, green, blue, indigo and violet. These types of tricks can really improve your memory.

235. Stop telling yourself you have a weak memory. When you say these things you begin to plant the thought in your mind and it becomes a reality. Remind yourself constantly that you have a great memory and you can remember anything as long as you put your mind to the task. You will see an improvement in your recall ability.

236. Losing those unpleasant or negative thoughts can improve a person's memory. It is scientifically proven that people who have negative thoughts or are suffering from extreme amounts of stress tend to have a compromised memory. Ask your doctor about ways to get rid of stress.

237. Most of us live in routines. Our lives are centered around having the same routine each day or each week. If we stray from that routine it can keep us from being able to remember things. Your routine is what is holding back your memory. Change how you do things each day to force your brain to develop new ways of remembering and sorting information.

238. If you are trying to remember some body of information, one of the best techniques for doing so is to try to teach it to someone else. Teaching concepts to another person actually improves understanding and recall for both the student and

the teacher. Even something as simple as reading out loud to someone else can help too.

239.   Sleep well for at least 7-8 hours a day. A sleep deprived body has diminished functions including problems with brain activities and memory. Studies show that inadequate sleep can cause difficulties in problem solving, critical thinking and studying. Sleeping is an unavoidable part of the learning process as it is necessary for memory consolidation.

240.   Feed your brain. Just like the body, the brain needs fuel. A healthy diet, including vegetables, fruits and plenty of whole grains, can help to boost your memory. In addition, try to limit saturated fat in your diet. Saturated fats can hinder concentration and memory. Drinking alcohol in moderation can also help your memory and cognitive skills. One glass of red wine a day is the ideal option.

241.   Jigsaw puzzles are good to improve your memory. Choose the harder ones (500-600 piece puzzles) for greater benefits. This game requires visual judgment, critical thinking and shifting focus from the small pieces to the big picture several times. Mastering your jigsaw puzzles skills will help you when you need to use your memory in your everyday life.

242.   Improving your memory may be something as simple as going out for a jog or a bike ride. Recent studies have shown that aerobic exercises can actually cause the development of new neurons in the hippocampus of the brain, which is considered to be the memory store center of the brain.

243.   A great tip that can help you improve your memory is to seek help if you're suffering from depression. Depression can do a number on your brain. It can make it hard for you to concentrate and remember things. Getting proper treatment can help you improve your memory.

244.   A great tip that can help you improve your memory is to make sure you're getting enough healthy fats in your diet that contain omega-3's. These healthy fats are great because they support brain health. You can find omega-3's in salmon, flaxseed, or you can just take a fish oil supplement.

245.   Cramming is a very poor way to study and should be avoided. If your goal is to store information in memory, you should schedule multiple sessions to study. Try not to learn and memorize things all at one time. Your mind will be overwhelmed, and you will not remember the information for very long. Make sure you study

regularly so that your brain is stimulated into remembering.

246.   If you are a student studying for a test, it is important not to over study. Of course it is natural to want to remember information on the test, but by studying too much you are actually overworking your brain cells, which in turn could cause you to not remember anything.

247.   If you need to remember an important amount of information, study it in different locations. This allows you to create a visual link with a set of information, making it easier to internalize. In other words, learning the material in different places encourages it to become a part of your long-term memory.

248.   In order to improve your memory, be sure that you exercise on a regular basis. It is proven that exercise makes a person more alert, which in turn, helps you to absorb and keep information in the mind. Also, when your mind is alert, it is easier for it to take mental pictures.

249.   Keep a diary or calendar for appointments. This is extremely helpful in remembering important dates or events. Be consistent with it and keep it in the same place all the time. You should look at it

every day to update it and to make sure there isn't anything you are forgetting.

250. If you notice that you are having trouble with your memory, you may want to try running or riding a bicycle on a regular basis. Medical research has shown that running and bicycle riding stimulates the growth of new brain cells, which in turn, helps to improve a person's memory.

251. When trying to remember something, having patience with yourself will help you greatly! The harder you try to think of something, the more stressed you become, and of course, the more stressed you become the more difficult it is to remember anything! Take a deep breath, relax, and try to clear your mind and before you know it what ever you were trying so hard to recall will pop right up in your mind!

252. It is important that you keep a daily routine if you want to improve your memory. By doing things at different times of the day, you may forget certain obligations. Try to stick with one routine for the weekdays when you are at work and one routine for weekends when you are home.

253. Feed your brain. Just like the body, the brain needs fuel. A healthy diet, including vegetables,

fruits and plenty of whole grains, can help to boost your memory. In addition, try to limit saturated fat in your diet. Saturated fats can hinder concentration and memory. Drinking alcohol in moderation can also help your memory and cognitive skills. One glass of red wine a day is the ideal option.

254.   Knowing what type of learner you are will enable you to reinforce your memory! If you know that you are a visual learner, for example, then keep a small notebook with you at all times to write down the information you need to remember, or if you are an auditory learner, use a small recorder. These small aids will be a big help when you need to call on your memory later!

255.   It may sound silly, but one way to improve memory is to surround yourself with good friends, and to maintain an active social life. A Harvard study suggests that those who had active and fulfilling social lives, showed rates of cognitive decline significantly lower than their less socially active peers.

256.   A good tip that can help you improve your memory is to make sure that you're keeping your stress levels in check. Too much stress has been shown to severely impair memory functions. Take

some time to relax and unwind if you are looking to improve your memory.

257.   Do not have any doubts about your memory. A lot of people assume that with age, your memory goes as well. However, this isn't always true. Anticipating memory loss can actually cause it. When people begin to doubt your mental acuity, it becomes easier to believe that about yourself. Believe in yourself and do not be so sensitive to what other people say.

258.   The next time your memory fails to help you remember where you placed something, be sure to jog your memory. Try to remember where you last placed something and how long ago it was. From now on, try to keep your items in the same place so you do not forget where they are.

259.   To remember things like turning off the water, place some object that will remind you in a place where you are likely to trip over it! If you have left the sprinklers on for half an hour while you go inside to eat, put your garden gloves in the kitchen sink or some other unlikely place. This will remind you to turn off the water!

260.   Memory is just like the muscles in your body, if you don't use it, you'll lose it. A way to keep your

memory active is to change up your brain's routine every so often. By doing the same activities over and over, you don't give your memory a chance to learn something new. By doing this, you will eventually start to lose your memory. Work your memory out by doing different activities including brain-stimulating activities in order to get the most out of your memory.

261.   The best way to improve your memory if you're studying, is to add structure to what you're attempting to learn. Categorizing and taking things one step at a time, will allow you to learn and to retain the knowledge of a previous subject, before you move on to the next. This is undoubtedly the best way to study.

262.   Like an actor does before putting on a play, rehearsing what you learn is a great way to improve your memory. If you are attempting to study, recite the problems and answers aloud, and you will absorb the information easier, and ultimately, retain it more efficiently. This is a great way to improve your overall memory.

263.   If you need to remember an important amount of information, study it in different locations. This allows you to create a visual link with a set of information, making it easier to internalize. When

you study the information in a variety of places, it is more likely to be stored in your long-term memory.

264.   Eat more onions to improve your memory. A few studies have isolated fisetin to be of great benefit in improving the long term memory. You can find beneficial levels of fisetin in onions, strawberries, mangos and other plants. It also is a strong antioxidant so it will deliver other benefits to your body as well.

265.   Feed your brain. Just like the body, the brain needs fuel. A healthy diet, including vegetables, fruits and plenty of whole grains, can help to boost your memory. In addition, try to limit saturated fat in your diet. Saturated fats can hinder concentration and memory. Drinking alcohol in moderation can also help your memory and cognitive skills. One glass of red wine a day is the ideal option.

266.   If you have a hard time memorizing things, it is wise to try not to learn too many new things at the same time. Wait until you have fully memorized a piece of information before moving on to the other. Learning many things at the same time will just make everything scramble in your brain.

267.   As if you needed another excuse to exercise, physical activity enhances the effects of helpful

chemicals within the brain and actually protects brain cells! Exercise is one potent weapon in improving your memory or maintaining more of it, as you get older. So keep active, keep moving and keep more in memory!

268.   A memory technique that works for many people is the listen, write and read method. Basically what this entails is really listening to what is being said. While listening, make notes about the material that is being shared. At a later time, read the notes again. With this technique, you are actually reviewing the information three times which aids in cementing the information in your memory.

269.   If you find that you are losing things as soon as you set them down, try dedicating a spot to them. Make sure that you are putting your keys in the same spot every day. Make a spot for your glasses or the book you are reading. If you make a habit of putting everything in its place, forgetting where they are won't be a problem.

270.   If you have a list of words that you need to remember, try putting them in alphabetical order. Our society has already categorized many common items into alphabetical lists, so it is a pattern that your brain is familiar with. As a result, when you alphabetize a list of words, your brain recognizes

the well-known familiar pattern and has an easier time recalling them at a later date.

271.   If you suffer from loss of memory, be sure to see a psychiatrist or therapist. Memory loss can be a sign that you suffer from anxiety or depression, and you may not even know it. If you do have anxiety or depression, treating it could be the key to you getting your memory back.

272.   Scent has a huge impact on memory. If you keep something that you enjoy smelling right next to where you keep things, you will have an easier time recalling where the object is. For example, if you keep a plug in air freshener right next to where you keep you wallet when you are home, you will have no problem remembering where it is.

273.   You can remember information more easily if you focus on it without distractions while studying. Humans need to store information in their long-term memory before they can easily remember it. It's hard to do this effectively if you have any other distractions at that time.

274.   A great way to improve your memory is a physical exercise While you typically think of physical exercise as good for the body, it's also an exceptional way to increase your memory. By

increasing the supply of oxygen to your brain, exercise helps reduce your risk for diseases and disorders that eventually lead to memory loss.

275.   Help protect your memory for years to come by making sure you are getting plenty of vitamin B-12 in your diet. Studies have linked low levels of B-12 to dementia and poor cognitive function. Food sources rich in B-12 include liver, eggs, fish, poultry, meat and milk products. If you don't eat a lot of meat, you may need to take a daily B-12 supplement to help prevent deficiency.

276.   Drink more milk for healthy brain activity for life. Milk is a veritable treasure trove of B vitamins, potassium, magnesium and calcium that all have incredibly important functions for taking care of your brain. These vitamins and minerals do a great job in supporting the functions of your brain. The healthier the brain, the better the memory will be.

277.   Make sure that your diet has good sources of Omega-3 fatty acids. Most commonly found in fish, these fatty acids do a superb job of keeping your brain on its toes. Numerous studies have shown a positive benefit to the brain when the diet contains omega-3's. Try adding pink salmon, walnuts and flax seed, so you can get this essential fat.

278.   After you learn something new, teach it to another person. When you teach it, it forces your brain to manipulate the information in another way in order for you to articulate it. This manipulation of information strengthens that part of your memory, and it is an effective way in committing the new information into your brain.

279.   To successfully remember information, you need to give it your complete and undivided attention. For information to move out of your short-term memory and into your long-term memory, you need to be carefully attending to it. Be sure that you read and study in a quiet place without any other distractions.

280.   Since repetition enforces memory, repeat important information over and over in your mind immediately after hearing or learning it. Be it the name of a new client or your wedding anniversary, by rehearsing information you will keep it fresh in your mind. Not only will this assist you in remembering the important details, but this is also a very useful exercise for your memory in general.

281.   In order to maintain a strong memory, be sure to remain active in a social context. Social interactions keep you alert and uplifted. Your brain cells will not get stimulated when you are feeling

lonely or depressed. Your mind stays strong when you are involved in stimulating conversations.

282.   Make your memorization easier by using mnemonic devices. The easiest one is to associate a visual image with the word or name you need to remember. Life like, vivid images linked to hard to memorize or understand concepts can help to speed up the learning process significantly. Think of images from your everyday life to make the process easier and faster.

283.   Use mnemonic devices to improve your memory. A mnemonic device is any rhyme, joke, song, or phrase that triggers memory of another fact, such as the abbreviation Roy G Biv, which tells you the colors of the spectrum. The best mnemonic devices are those which use humor or positive imagery, as you will have an easier time remembering them.

284.   Try to memorize things in sets of 7. According to studies, the human capacity for Short Term Memory, or (STM) is 7, add or minus 2. This is why humans memorize things best in groups of 7. This is also why, for example, your phone number is seven digits.

285.   Use a mnemonic device to help yourself remember things. Create a picture in your head in relation to what you anticipate needing to remember. You can work it into an unusual sentence or make it into a fun acronym. Mnemonic devices are much easier for the brain to remember than straight facts.

286.   Establish relationships with old and new information. To keep your memory in top form, keep information relevant in your mind. Your brain will automatically discard most facts it deems useless. It is often necessary to "update" memories. Think on them regularly and determine how they relate or hold up to new information.

287.   Many people use visualization to remember information. Try visualizing what you wish to remember, create mind pictures, draw diagrams or charts to aid in remembering information in textbooks or during lectures at school. The mind is very effective in remembering visual details and recalling images, even images long-forgotten.

288.   A good way to remember names and improve memory is to use pictures to associate with the names. If the persons name is Bob Frost, try to remember them covered in frost. If the persons name is Gemma Hand, try to picture them standing

and applauding giving someone standing ovation or giving them a hand moving.

289.   One way to improve your memory is by adding meditation to your daily routine. Meditating helps to relax your mind and body, which in turn can make it easier for your brain to recall memories. Set aside a specific time each day when you know you won't be interrupted to close your eyes and meditate for as long as you would like.

290.   Exercise your brain. Using your memory and other thought provoking functions of your brain daily, will help keep your mind and your memory sharp. Do puzzles, drive a different way to work and memorize something every day. You will see an improvement quickly and less of a decline as time moves on.

291.   Keep a running list of the things you want to accomplish each day. As you finish one item, cross it off and move on to the next. Simultaneously, keep adding items at the bottom of the list as they arise. In this way you will never forget what you need to do next.

292.   If you are searching for ways to increase your memory, then work with others and collaborate on ideas with them. When you do this, your brain fires

in a different way than it does when you work on something alone. Bounce ideas off others and see how differently you begin to think.

293.   It is important to get a sufficient amount of sleep if you are trying to improve your memory. Medical studies have shown that getting enough sleep every night can improve both short and long term memory. Your brain cannot absorb new information when your body has not gotten a lot of sleep.

294.   To help yourself remember something jot down some notes, say them aloud and keep your notes organized. When you involve different functions of your body such as writing and talking to remember something, those physical activities will help your brain recall more effectively. In addition, the notes serve as a visual memory aid.

295.   Learning doesn't end once you have your college diploma, so commit to lifelong learning. When you don't learn anything new, the part of your brain that controls memory isn't being used. Then, when you have to recall something, you might discover that it is difficult for you.

296.   When you're having trouble remembering something, like when you've been studying for too

long and can't focus on the information anymore, try getting outside and taking a walk or jog. This will help you clear your head and get more oxygen pumping to your brain, thus letting your brain work at a higher capacity.

297.   Pay attention to the environments that pop up in your memories. These locations may enhance your learning abilities. Return to these types of locations, or replicate their effects, in order to bring about the memory-enhancing effect of those places. Many people find that a certain level of background noise, for example, is vital to their learning.

298.   Sleep at least eight hours per night. Research indicates that not sleeping enough will affect your ability to remember things on a daily basis. Concentration is needed to push current events over to long-term memory.

299.   Before you make a commitment to improve your memory, be sure you are all ready to do so and keep an open mind. Some people's memories will not improve because they are not willing to try certain techniques given to them. Tell yourself that with enough hard work, your memory will work fine in no time!

300.   Keep your self organized. It is important that you don't waste your time trying to remember simple things, like where you put your car keys. Just make sure to keep them in the same spot every day until it becomes habbit. Being organized will actually work to enhance your memory.

301.   If someone you know is suffering from Dementia, Alzheimer's Disease, or another illness that effects their memory, try showing them pleasant pictures from the past. By looking at pleasant memories, the memory of these patients may improve. Be sure not to bring up unpleasant memories as this could cause them a setback.

302.   Adding fish oil to your diet can boost your memory. Research has proven that the omega-3 fatty acids found in these oils are beneficial for the memory. It's crucial that you receive the right dosage. Therefore, you should get in touch with your physician prior to taking this supplement.

303.   Things are easier to remember if they have a special meaning to you. Think about why you need to memorize the information. For example, if you are going shopping, ask yourself why. It could be for your child's birthday and thinking about that, will help you remember what you need to buy.

304.   If you are attempting to learn new material, try teaching it to someone else. Talking through concepts and ideas will help you remember the material. Trying to explain it to another person will increase your understanding of the terms and you are also more likely to remember it. Pair up with another student in your class and use this technique to help you study.

305.   If you have trouble remembering things, don't be afraid to take notes, make lists or use a day planner to keep track of your schedule. These helpful tools can take some of the stress out of trying to remember everything on your own. Once you have lowered your stress levels by writing everything down, you may even find that your memory improves, since too much stress can inhibit memory.

306.   Have you ever put down something somewhere and then later couldn't remember where it was? In order to help your brain with memory retention try setting things down and saying aloud to yourself what you are doing, such as "I am putting the keys on the top of my dresser in my bedroom." The effort of stating the sentence aloud will help your brain to retrace that memory later when you need to find your keys.

307.   A lot of the information we learn is very close to information we already know, so improving your memory can be as simple as playing an association game. Make sure that anything new you're attempting to learn can tie in with someone you already know, and you will develop smooth transitions between one piece of material and the next.

308.   Make sure your attention if focused on the material you want to remember. If you have other distractions going on around you - music playing, the TV on, kids talking, etc. - your mind won't be able to focus on the material. This will result in it being hard to remember what you've studied.

309.   A good way to help you remember things is to keep repeating them outloud. Eventually, this information is going to be embedded into your head if you keep hearing it over and over again. For instance, if you have to clean your room on Saturday, keep saying so outloud.

310.   Avoid smoking cigarettes to keep your memory from being negatively affected. Studies have shown that the memory of smokers suffers more than compared to non-smokers. You probably didn't need yet another reason to quit, but maybe this will be the one that lets you finally put down that pack.

311.   One way to improve your memory is by limiting distractions and focusing only on the information you want to remember. With today's hectic lifestyle, most people spend a great deal of time multitasking. By clearing all distractions and focusing only on the information you are trying to remember, it allows you to build a strong, clear memory that will be easy to recall at a later time.

312.   It is crucial that you eat breakfast if you are trying to improve your memory. Many doctors and health professionals have found that eating breakfast fuels the mind after not having eaten for many hours because of sleep. Even if it is a bowl of fruit, be sure to never skip breakfast.

313.   The best way to keep your memory sharp is to make sure that you stay mentally active. Physical exercise keeps your body in shape, and mental exercise keeps your mind in shape. Doing crossword puzzles, reading complicated passages, playing board games, or learning a musical instrument can all help you keep your mental edge.

314.   Many people suggest creating relationships between a new concept or image and an amusing phrase or picture. This type of creative thinking makes it easier to store new information for later

access. Using a funny mnemonic device creates a humorous, entertaining association with the piece of information, and you will be able to recall it more easily in the future.

315.   Here is food for "thought!"□ Consume food known to enhance brain functions. Omega-3 fatty acids, fruits and vegetables are known to provide the necessary nutrients for improved memory. Avoid eating fatty, heavy dishes; limit the intake of saturated fat and consider spring water instead of wine or beer. Eat considerable amounts of whole grains to avoid the early onset of Dementia.

316.   If you are finding your memory is lacking it may be because of a lack of sleep. As such try getting more rest. Scientists believe that when we are asleep it is when our brain sorts through the events of our lives and files them away, like a librarian and a filing cabinet. They also believe this is why we dream.

317.   Avoid cramming. Work in regular study sessions that you have set out on a schedule. Having a set time to study will help your brain remember the facts you present to it. Cramming simply presents your brain with too much information to remember at any one time, and so you will forget much of it.

318.   A good tip that can help you improve your memory is to participate in activities that can challenge you mentally. When it comes to memory, if you don't use it, you lose it. Pick an activity you're not familiar with so that it's a good challenge for you.

319.   To help a young child remember his home phone number, use a familiar tune and make up a song with the phone number. When the phone number is associated with the familiarity of the tune, the child will be able to recall the phone number a lot better. This method is useful for people of any age.

320.   If you have forgotten something important that you need to remember, close your eyes and take a deep breath. Try breathing exercises by holding your breath in for a few seconds and releasing it. After doing this a few times, go back to trying to remember what you have forgotten.

321.   Do not cram information before an exam or a test. You will remember better if you study regularly. You can improve your memory by making it work on a regular basis, and you will remember something more easily if you go over it everyday instead of focusing on it for a few hours only.

322.   Try to study beyond what you really need to know. In-depth knowledge of a given topic facilitates easier recall. For example, if you want to know the meaning of a word, you should read all about it.

323.   When trying to commit an item such as study materials to memory, it is best that you focus on these in an environment which is free from distractions such as television or music. Items can only move from the short term memory into the long term memory if you actively pay attention to the topic on hand.

324.   Try learning a new language. Learning a new language can really help to keep your mind and memory in shape. It has also been proven to delay brain deterioration and dementia. Just immersing yourself in the language will do. There is no need to become a fluent speaker of it.